Cool Recipes for HOT WOMEN

HOW TO EAT YOUR WAY TO A HEALTHY MENOPAUSE

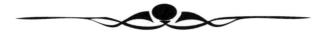

PAT DUCKWORTH

www.hotwomencoolsolutions.com

JENNY TSCHIESCHE

www.jennytschiesche.com

Published by
HWCS Publications
White House, Meeting Lane
Litlington
Royston, Cambs
England SG8 0QF

Goran Cover design
Visualarts

Rebecca Dandy Editor

Ginger Marks Layout
DocUmeantDesigns

www.DocUmeantDesigns.com

For inquiries about volume orders, please contact the publisher in writing.

Printed in The United Kingdom
ISBN-13: 978-0-9926620-1-1
ISBN-10: 0-9926620-1-X

CONTENTS

ACKNOWLEDGMENTS

I am grateful to my 'Book Family' for all of their love, help and support. Particularly Marina Nani, Kim Bridge-Wright, John Bridge-Wright, Danielle Serpico, Annie Newman, Serah Lister and Jonna Tuomola.

A special thanks to my friend Jenny Tschiesche for being my partner in this project.

FOREWORD

I got to know Pat Duckworth when she interviewed me in connection with her first book, 'Hot Women, Cool Solutions'. Not only was it great fun, but I was impressed by her holistic approach to helping women get their menopause symptoms under control. I found Pat's enthusiasm and energy about bringing her knowledge and ideas to women on both sides of the Atlantic exciting.

Expanding on the guidance about nutrition included in that book, she has joined forces with leading UK nutritionist, Jenny Tschiesche. Together, they provide a delicious array of recipes to put the principles of eating your way to a healthy menopause into practice. It's about a truly satisfying way of savouring good, healthy food and learning about new ingredients to enjoy.

If you wonder how much what you eat and drink can affect your menopause symptoms, Pat will help you to identify your triggers and discover the foods that will support you. As a contemporary and as a therapist who has helped many women, Pat understands and fully embraces the fact that we are all different and our experiences during this stage of life are unique. However, there are some popular foods and ingredients that may be aggravating your symptoms.

This is about much more than hot flashes. As the balance of your hormones change, there is an impact on your heart, digestion, bones, skin, hair and nails—in fact your whole body. Knowing the right things to eat is essential if you want to nourish your body through menopause and life after menopause. Your post-menopause life could be as long as 30 or 40 years. I want to be as fit as possible to enjoy that time. In fact, I want it to be the best time possible.

I enjoy food and have always thought of myself as a healthy eater, but it is easy to forget the connection between the food you eat and the symptoms you experience. Starting the journey through menopause is a chance to reassess your eating habits and make changes to support your physical, emotional and mental health. Let's do it!

Susie Hadas, Founder & CEO
Personally Cool Inc.
www.mycoldfront.com

INTRODUCTION

As I approached my mid-50s I was feeling pretty good. I had not started to experience menopause symptoms, my weight was steady and my BMI was around 20. All around me my female friends were fanning themselves and complaining about their thickening waists. And then suddenly my periods became irregular, my weight went up by half a stone and I had my first hot flush.

A few months and many hot flushes later, I went to Japan for a once-in-a-lifetime holiday. I was staying in traditional Japanese hotels, eating local foods and drinking green tea. And guess what? The hot flushes disappeared completely. I returned home and went back to my usual diet, which I have always considered to be relatively healthy. Within a few days the hot flushes were back.

There were a number of factors involved in this experience. Firstly, I was on holiday and therefore relaxed. Secondly, I was sightseeing and spending a major part of each day walking around and getting lots of exercise. Thirdly, it was November and the ambient temperature was comfortably cool. And lastly, and most importantly,

I had eliminated or reduced a lot of food triggers from my diet including red meat, spices, chocolate, wine and caffeine.

As a therapist, when I work with women who are experiencing menopause symptoms, the first thing I want to understand is what triggers their symptoms. This could be something in their environment, it could be something to do with their lifestyle but it is often something to do with what they are eating or drinking.

It is easy to become dissociated from noticing the effects of food on your body. You might not even have noticed a pattern of what you are consuming and the response from your body. In the first part of this book you will discover more about:

- symptoms and potential triggers
- symptom reducers
- the role of food supplements and
- maintaining a healthy weight

The recipes in this book are not just for women who are experiencing menopause symptoms as a natural stage in their lives. It will also help if your menopause symptoms are related to medical interventions such as hysterectomy, radiotherapy or hormone treatment for breast cancer.

I really hope you find this book informative.

Warm regards,
Pat, April 2014

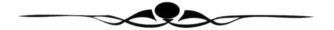

Why write a menopause cookery book?

We know there is a link between the food we eat and our overall health. In fact Hippocrates himself said, "Let food be thy medicine and let thy medicine be food". However, there's an abundance of theory and fact about what we should be eating to get a particular health benefit or outcome. There's also an abundance of cookery books and increasingly cookery shows on the television. However, these two worlds rarely come together.

As a nutrition expert with a passion for food it is my job to make theory a reality. I am Jenny Tschiesche, also known as the Lunchbox Doctor. I studied nutrition at the Institute of Optimum Nutrition from 2003-2009. When I graduated with my nutrition degree I wanted to make a difference to the general public's perception of healthy eating.

Healthy eating doesn't have to be boring; it doesn't have to lack flavour. I have been fortunate to work with a number of Michelin starred chefs and I have learned from their knowledge of what pleases palates and what looks good on a plate (though I will never claim to be 'chef' material in this department). I am an experienced home cook and tutor and I am passionate about food.

Happy cooking!
Jenny, April 2014

CHAPTER 1

WHAT IS MY BODY PLAYING AT?

The term 'menopause' is often used to refer to the years of women's lives either side of their last menstrual period. It is sometimes called 'the change' or 'time of life'. More technically correct terms are defined below.

Menopause can occur as early as 45 or not until 55 but the average age in the UK is 52 and 51 in the USA. You can also start to experience menopausal symptoms earlier as you enter into the 'perimenopause'.

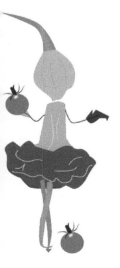

Menopause that occurs before the age of 40 is known medically as premature ovarian failure or POF. This occurs in 1 to 4 per cent of women. Early menopause can be precipitated by illnesses and medical interventions

Including radiotherapy and hysterectomy, but in up to 70 per cent of cases there is no obvious medical reason. In these cases it is advisable to seek medical investigation.

Definitions

Various terms are used in connection with menopause and some of them can be a bit confusing. It is useful to understand what is generally meant by these terms, particularly if you want to talk to health professionals

Pre-menopause—the early years of the transition period when menstrual periods may become irregular and sometimes heavier. Other menopause symptoms may be experienced. Generally, this stage starts after the age of 40.

Perimenopause—this is the stage either side of your last menstrual period when you notice most physical changes and when periods may become more irregular before they finally stop.

Menopause—your last menstrual period. You will only know that this was your last period when you have not had a menstrual bleed for 12 months.

Post-menopause—this relates to the years after your last period up to the end of your life. It overlaps with the perimenopause.

Andropause—the male menopause. Men produce less testosterone after the age of 40. This can lead to fewer and harder to sustain erections, hot flushes, lethargy, mood swings, irritability, and decreased sexual desire.

This book will help you to eat well all through perimenopause.

Symptoms of perimenopause can include:

- Tension
- Mood swings
- Depression
- Forgetfulness
- Poor or interrupted sleep
- Weight change
- Headache
- Tiredness
- Dizziness or faintness
- Heart pounding
- Hot flushes
- Night sweats
- Irregular periods
- Heavier/lighter periods
- Breast tenderness
- Abdominal bloating

Some women experience minimal symptoms but other women experience frequent and intense symptoms, which can disrupt their lives. Whichever category you are in, it is important to eat well and maintain a healthy weight.

Body changes

Just as during puberty, hormonal changes during perimenopause bring about changes to your weight and body shape. At this stage of your life, your metabolism will be slowing down and you may be naturally losing muscle which helps you to burn off fat.

During this phase of your life your ovaries produce less oestrogen and your body tries to compensate by manufacturing oestrogen elsewhere to protect your body against osteoporosis. The fat around the middle of your body is one of the sites where oestrogen is produced. So a little bit of weight gain around your waist is not your body turning against you—it's trying to look after you!

Strategies that you have used in the past to lose weight may not work as well now. Calorie controlled diets are not the answer. Diets make your body think that you are being starved and as soon as you eat normally again, it will replenish the fat stores in case there is a famine again. A better approach is about a long-term, different relationship to food.

It is useful to keep a Food Journal to help you to identify any patterns of how, when, and what you eat. We have made available to you a downloadable journal at www.hotwomencoolsolutions.com.

Apples Vs Pears

Gaining weight around the waist and changing to an 'apple' shape may be among the first signs of peri-menopause for some women. Alternatively, you may put weight on around your hips and thighs giving rise to the 'pear' shape.

As explained above, a small amount of weight gain around your middle is ok. However, excessive fat in that area can be a sign of stress and can be dangerous for your health and particularly your risk of breast cancer (Glenville, 2006).

The time to take action is if your waist to hip ratio exceeds 0.8. To calculate this, measure your waist and hips and then divide your waist measurement by your hip measurement. If your ratio is higher than 0.8 it can increase your risk of a range of conditions including cancer, high blood pressure, and stroke.

The 'Mindful Eating' advice in Chapter 3 applies to apples and pears.

Underweight

This is not about being naturally slim or thin, this is about your weight being too low to support your health and wellbeing. Being underweight is an issue at any stage of a woman's life. When you are younger if you are underweight it can affect your periods and your fertility. During perimenopause it can increase your risk of osteoporosis.

If you are generally eating well and you are losing weight you should seek advice from your doctor. It can be a sign of an overactive thyroid or coeliac disease.

Foods that trigger symptoms

These days we have become disconnected from the effects of food on our bodies. Women will often be aware of the foods that lead to weight gain but be less aware of the foods that change their mood, lead to hot flushes or cause changes to their skin.

Every woman is different and the foods that trigger symptoms will vary from person to person but there are some common triggers. The first stage in understanding your triggers is to keep a Symptom Journal (see Appendix A). That will help you to identify patterns of symptoms, environmental factors and food.

Common triggers for hot flushes include:

- Hot food and drinks that raise the body's base temperature

- Spicy foods
- Red meat
- Red wine
- Chocolate
- Coffee
- Fizzy drinks

There are some foods that are not beneficial to women at this stage of life. It may be difficult to eliminate them from your life completely but you will experience positive effects from reducing your intake.

1.   Refined carbohydrates

- Carbohydrates are sugar and starches and they are an important part of your diet as they give you energy. The most important thing to consider is whether they are refined or unrefined. Refined carbohydrates have the fibre and the nutritional goodness stripped away. This means that when you eat them glucose will be released into your bloodstream quickly causing a sugar spike and your body responds by producing insulin. The higher your blood sugar goes up, the lower it crashes down. When it crashes, your body will demand a quick sugar fix and it will release the stress hormones adrenaline and cortisol into your system.

- Refined carbohydrates include brown and white sugar, white flour, white pasta and breakfast cereals (including 'instant' porridge)
- Refined sugar is empty calories, it has no nutritional value. It boosts the feel good hormone serotonin but the effect is short-lived. Unlike other foods, sugar does not trigger a signal to the brain that you are full-up so there is no signal to the body to stop eating it.
- There are many negative effects on your physical and emotional health from eating refined carbohydrates. These include: tiredness, mood swings, anxiety and tension, Inability to concentrate, headaches, dizziness, palpitations, forgetfulness, weight gain—especially around the waist, lack of sex drive, high cholesterol, thyroid problems, risk of Type 2 diabetes and feeling more stressed

2. Caffeine

- Caffeine has many effects on the body. It is a stimulant that activates the adrenal glands. Caffeine blocks the brain chemical, adenosine, which slows us down and makes us sleep. It raises levels of dopamine and serotonin, keeping us alert but disrupting normal sleep patterns.

- Caffeine is present in varying quantities in coffee, tea, chocolate, cola drinks and energy drinks. It is also present in some medications.
- Caffeine causes a quick rise in blood sugar which can affect your energy and your moods. It can cause the blood vessels to expand making you sweat more which can increase hot flushes. It has a diuretic effect which means that you can lose important vitamins and minerals. The acidic effect of caffeine on the body means that calcium will be lost through your urine.
- Caffeine has an addictive effect on the body and it is better to wean yourself off slowly. Try drinking green tea, white tea, herb tea or rooibos which naturally grows without caffeine

3.   Dairy Products

- The consumption of dairy products is usually associated with bone health. Milk and dairy products contain calcium, phosphorous, magnesium and protein.
- In modern dairy farms, cows are milked for about 300 days a year and for much of that time, the cows are pregnant. The milk from a cow in the late stage of pregnancy contains much higher amounts of an oestrogen compound, oestrone sulphate. Most cow's milk

also contains measurable amounts of antibiotics, herbicides and pesticides.

- Dairy products contain the protein casein which many people find difficult to digest. This can lead to lack of energy and is linked to allergic reactions.
- Dairy products can lead to the production of excess mucous in the respiratory system, giving rise to nasal congestion, catarrh and a phlegm in the throat

4.   Alcohol

- Alcohol is both a stimulant and a depressant. It contains sugar which goes straight into the blood stream having a disruptive effect on your blood sugar levels
- Alcohol has a diuretic effect and can lead to dehydration. It blocks the effect of some valuable nutrients such as vitamin B. zinc, calcium and magnesium and essential fatty acids.
- Alcohol effects the functioning of your liver which is important during menopause because your liver controls the amount of oestrogen circulating in your blood.
- Drinking alcohol at night can have a disruptive effect on your sleep pattern

5.   Cigarettes

- I know they are not a food but it would be wrong not to mention the effect of cigarettes.
- Nicotine stimulates adrenaline to release sugar into the bloodstream giving you a sugar peak. This is followed by a drop which is associated with a drop in mood.
- Smoking cigarettes depletes the body of nutrients such as vitamin C, reducing your energy and your immune system. The negative health effects of nicotine include increased risk of heart disease, lung cancer, stroke, emphysema and hypertension.

As a final point in this section, be aware of xenoestrogens in your environment and take action to avoid ingesting them. These are common chemical ingredients found in pesticides and many plastic products including food containers and wrappings. Once they are inside the bloodstream they mimic the action of oestrogen. To reduce your intake of xenoestrogens, eat organic foods wherever possible and never heat up food in a plastic container in the microwave

For your Bonus Gifts go to
www.hotwomencoolsolutions.com

CHAPTER 2

WHAT CAN I EAT TO HELP WITH MY SYMPTOMS?

Nutrition is defined as: "The act or process of nourishing or being nourished; specifically: the sum of the processes by which an animal or plant takes in and utilizes food substances. Inadequate nutrient intake or absorption leads to malnutrition and disease." (Merriam-Webster Dictionary)

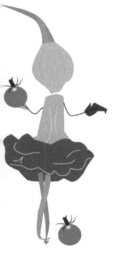

Good nutrition is about fuelling our bodies in a way that helps it to function effectively and efficiently.

Some general food guidelines:

Eat simple, unprocessed foods whenever possible so that you know exactly what you are eating. Avoid processed foods, low fat and diet products that often contain preservatives, salt and added sugar.

Eat organic where practicable. Some fruit and vegetables are more prone to having pesticides on their skin than others. These are: apples, bell peppers, celery, cherries, grapes, nectarines, peaches, pears, raspberries, spinach and strawberries.

Start the day with breakfast—people who do find it easier to lose weight. Eating protein at breakfast will keep you feeling fuller for longer.

Keep your diet healthy, balanced and satisfying.

If you want to lose weight, eat vegetables that grow above ground—they store less sugar.

Watch your portion size—reducing the size of your plate will reduce your food intake.

Don't skip meals. If you let yourself get too hungry you are more likely to eat carbohydrates.

Make sure you drink enough—preferably water or cool, non-caffeine drinks.

Nutrition for a Healthy Menopause

1. Phytoestrogens are oestrogen hormone-like compounds that can help to balance your hormones and

reduce hot flushes and night sweats. They are naturally occurring in plant foods and readily absorbed in the digestive system. They include:

- Isoflavones—found in soy (tofu, miso and tempeh), chickpeas, lentils and kidney beans. Eat a variety of these foods in order to get a balance of isoflavones. The best foods for breast health* are tofu and miso (Glenville 1997).

- Lignans—found in flaxseeds (linseeds), sesame seeds, sunflower seeds, brown rice, oats, broccoli and carrots. Lignans have a balancing effect on oestrogen and the fibre content helps to remove excess oestrogens through the bowels.

- Coumestans—found in split peas, pinto beans, lima beans, sprouted mung beans and alfalfa beans.

2. Omega-3 fatty acids are found in sardines, salmon, mackerel and flaxseeds (linseeds). When you eat foods containing omega-3, your body produces prostaglandins which are anti-inflammatory. These substances are essential for healthy skin, joints, thyroid, weight control, lower blood pressure and reducing the risk of cardiovascular disease.

3. Omega-6 fatty acids are found in nuts, seeds and legumes. They can be converted into either anti-inflammatory or pro-inflammatory prostaglandins. You need some of the inflammatory prostaglandins as they mobilise your immune system to deal with damage from bacterial attack or traumas such as cuts and bruises. However, excessive levels of omega-6

can cause inflammation of joints and skin. Therefore, it is important to have more omega-3 foods than omega-6 foods.

4. Carotenoids are found in dark and orange-coloured fruits and vegetables such as carrots, sweet potatoes, tomatoes, pumpkin, cantaloupe, apricots, spinach and broccoli. They act as antioxidants that help to prevent damage to the cells in your body. Some carotenoids can be converted into vitamin A, which helps to maintain healthy skin, teeth, skeletal tissue and mucous membranes.

5. Unrefined carbohydrates come in 2 types: complex carbohydrates such as grains, beans, pulses, and vegetables; and simple carbohydrates such as fruit and honey. Unrefined carbohydrates provide valuable nutrients and a supply of slow-release energy. This enables you to avoid sugar surges and mood swings. This also supports the functioning of your adrenal glands that produce a form of oestrogen to help protect your bones.

6. Healthy fats are essential to the health of your body and your brain. Fat makes our food palatable and 'low-fat' or 'reduced fat' products often have sugar added in order to make them edible. Your diet should contain 'good' fats, which are found in lean meat, poultry, eggs, coconut oil, avocados and olive oil.

7. Water comes from the foods you eat as well as what you drink. Water-rich foods include iceberg lettuce, watermelon, broccoli, carrots, beets, oranges, apples,

bananas and sweetcorn. Your body is around 60 per cent water and you need water to transport nutrients around your body and to eliminate toxins. The effects of dehydration on the body are stress, headaches, back pain, high blood pressure and possible weight gain.

There is some debate about the right amount of water your body needs daily and it will depend on what you are eating and drinking and how much you are exercising. The usual recommendation is 2½ pints or 1.5 litres a day. You can take in water from tea and coffee but the caffeine in those drinks also dehydrates your body. It is best to drink water and non-caffeinated herb and fruit teas. Starting the day with a cup of hot water with a slice of lemon starts the rehydration process and helps to alkalise your stomach.

*Medical advice used to be that you should avoid phytoestrogens if you have been diagnosed with oestrogen receptor-positive breast cancer. However, current advice is that phytoestrogens may be beneficial but more research is required. Women in this situation can include phytoestrogens in their diet but should avoid phytoestrogen tablets (Goldman, 2010).

Food Supplements

You may be wondering whether you need to take food supplements if you are eating a healthy, balanced diet. If you are eating a good variety of food and you are still experiencing symptoms then you may require food supplements. Most vitamins and minerals are dependent on each other to work effectively so it is best to take a multi-vitamin and mineral supplement especially designed for menopause. You get what you pay for with food supplements and it is best to buy specialist menopause products. For suppliers, see the Resources section in Appendix D.

For your Bonus Gifts go to
www.hotwomencoolsolutions.com

CHAPTER 3

HOW DO I CONTROL MY WEIGHT?

If you want to lose weight or maintain a healthy weight, the first step is to understand the difference between physical and emotional hunger and only eat when you are physically hungry.

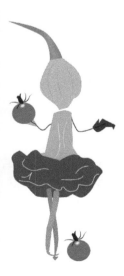

Physical hunger comes on slowly. You might gradually feel loss of energy, loss of concentration, irritable, lightheaded, empty, hunger pangs in stomach and, finally, must eat now! If you eat something when you are physically hungry, the hunger indicators will gradually fade away.

Emotional hunger comes on suddenly. You might start to salivate because you saw or smelled food, get the oral urge to chew or search through the cupboards to find something to satisfy a craving or feel sadness, anger or frustration. If you eat when you are emotionally hungry, you are likely to feel unsatisfied and possibly even sick.

If you start to eat before you're physically hungry you won't know when to stop eating. Also, if you do not eat when you start to feel hungry you are more likely to start to crave carbohydrates. When you are starving hungry, a salad doesn't look that appealing whereas a baguette or a sticky bun looks just right. Therefore, being aware of your current level of hunger is important

The signals for thirst and hunger are very similar so, if you start to feel hungry, have a drink of water and then wait for 10 minutes to feel if the hunger signal is still there. If it is, go ahead and eat.

The second step to losing or maintaining weight is to stop eating when you are satisfied. Do not wait for the 'full' or 'stuffed' signal as you will have eaten too much. There are 2 hormones that play an important role in regulating appetite and weight, 'ghrelin' and 'leptin'.

Ghrelin is produced by the stomach and it sends the message that you need to eat. Ghrelin levels fall when the food you eat arrives at your intestines. If you go on an extreme diet, more ghrelin gets secreted and your ability to burn calories starts to diminish.

Leptin is a hormone secreted by fat cells which regulates appetite and metabolism. Levels of leptin rise as we eat so that the appetite is suppressed. It also promotes calorie burning.

The levels of leptin and ghrelin can also be affected by your sleep patterns. Studies have found that people who regularly slept for just 5 hours a night had 15 per cent more ghrelin in their system, leading to feelings of hunger. They also had significantly less leptin to suppress the appetite. In light of this research, it is important to sort out any sleep issues before you try to lose weight.

The secret to recognising these signals and having time to react to them is to eat mindfully, that is:

- Sit down when you eat—even if it's only a snack.
- Take time to enjoy your food—look at, smell and taste the food.
- Slow down—put the knife and fork down between mouthfuls.
- Chew your food completely.
- Drink before you eat not while you are eating—if you drink while you are eating it may make it difficult to identify the signals for satisfaction.

- Concentrate on eating—don't do anything but eat; no television, radio, texting or reading.

Eating out can be a real challenge when you are establishing new eating habits and trying to lose weight. This can be a particular problem if alcohol is involved as you can tend to make unwise decisions and overeat after a few drinks.

When you are eating socially what's important isn't the food—it's the company. The problem is that when you are chatting with your friends you can lose track of what you are eating and how you are eating it.

Whether you are eating in a restaurant or at a dinner party keep to the same guidelines for mindful eating, that is, eat slowly and stop eating as soon as you are satisfied. Here are some more tips:

- Push the bread basket away and resist the temptation to eat before your meal starts by sipping water and chatting to your companions.
- Don't over order or overload your plate. You may be able to order 2 starters instead of a starter and a main course.
- You don't have to eat everything on your plate. If it really upsets you to leave food on your plate in a restaurant ask for a doggie bag. At dinner parties just say, "That was great, I'm really full."
- Ask for sauce or gravy on the side so that you can have a smaller amount.

- Trade potatoes for an extra vegetable that you enjoy.
- If you want a dessert, share one with a friend.

You can download a relaxation/hypnotic recording to help to support your weight loss at www.hotwomencoolsolutions.com

CHAPTER 4

FOOD FOR MENOPAUSE GUIDELINES

This chapter introduces you to some of the key concepts of eating for the Menopause. It provides an explanation for some of the more commonly available foodstuffs and also some of the less well known but increasingly available foodstuffs which make healthy eating more easy now than ever before. We shall be covering the different options for dairy and non-dairy milks, different types of flours and baking products, the options for using different sugars as well as the variety of soy sauces now available.

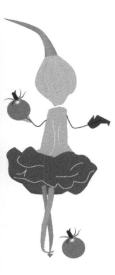

Dairy

As Pat mentioned earlier, there is a protein in dairy products called casein that isn't easily absorbed by the body. As a result, it can remain in the gut, undigested, where it may ferment and produce toxins and mucus that can stop the absorption of nutrients. It is important to reiterate this because over and over again dairy is touted as the prime source of calcium. However, it may not suit everyone. In fact increasingly it suits less and less people and there are better options even within the dairy food category to choose. Read on.

Cow-based dairy products are acid-forming. See the chart below.

Highly Alkalising	←		Natural or Almost Neutral		→	Highly Acid-Forming
Green vegetables and lettuce. Most vegetables Garlic, fennel, ginger Sea vegetables Sweet potatoes Sprouted seeds, grains and beans Tomatoes Avocado Lemons Sea salt	Raw almonds, Brazil nuts, burdock root, flax seed oil (linseed oil), raw sunflower seeds, fresh herbs, stevia.	Most fruit, cold pressed oils, raw carob	Raw honey, sprouted lentils, raw goat cheese (not pasteurised) and free from antibiotics and hormones)	Agave, brown rice syrup, olives, pasteurised soft goat cheese, cream, dates, sprouted grains, wild salmon, oysters	Meat, bacon, chicken, white rice, shrimp, turkey, veal, peanuts	Alcohol (all types), cola, coffee, non-herbal teas, pasteurised milk, ice cream, candy, sugar, artificial sweetners. Hydrogenated oils, fried and processed foods. Chocolate Margerine Jelly Stress Negativity Medication Hormone pills

Source: www.diaryofanutritionist.com

The problem with consuming too many acidic foods is that the body will attempt to purge the blood by leaching alkaline minerals (like calcium) directly from the bones, tissues and teeth. Unfortunately, this is at a time when reduced oestrogen levels lead to a natural level of bone loss anyway.

So in the recipes that follow, you will find a reduced amount of dairy but a prioritisation of goats and sheep based dairy products where dairy is used.

If you want to try some alternative non-dairy milk then here's a useful comparison.

Almond Milk has a great flavour and creaminess. This milk works in hot drinks (even in Rooibos tea) although your tea or coffee will be darker in colour with this milk versus cow's milk.

Coconut Milk is fantastic for cooking with.

Rice Milk has a lovely sweet flavour. It works very well in porridge but not so well in hot drinks as it separates.

Soy is similar to traditional milk when it comes to protein and calcium, however soy is another food allergen that may not agree with your body. It is also a controversial food where various studies show that soy milk may not be as good for us as we think for various reasons but including the phytates which may bind to other nutrients in our diet meaning we are less able to absorb those nutrients.

Milk/Properties	Almond*	Coconut	Rice	Soy*
Calories	Low	Low	High	Low
Protein	Low	Low	Low	High
Calcium	Similar To Dairy	Low	Low	Similar To Dairy
Sugars	Low	Low	High	Low

* The 'no added sugar' versions are low in both calories and sugars

Red Meat

Within this recipe book you will notice there are very few recommendations for red meat. Like cow's milk dairy products, red meat can also cause calcium to be leached from your bones due to the acidic effect it has on your body. A little is not going to harm you but eating red meat regularly can hinder your chances of reducing bone loss.

Flours

Both spelt and kamut flours are more easily tolerated than wheat. They both contain gluten. However because they are more easily tolerated and can be used fairly interchangeably (you may need to add a little more liquid with both if replacing wheat flour with either) they are recommended. Both are available at supermarkets. Spelt is more commonly available. Kamut can be found in health food stores also.

For gluten free flours try buckwheat, quinoa or millet flour. They are all nutritious and can provide a really good alternative to wheat flour. Using non-gluten flours however will necessitate the use of binders such as, xanthan gum, flaxseed or chia seeds, and eggs.

If you choose gluten free flours then you can also opt for gluten free baking powder which is also available in supermarkets in the 'Free From' section.

Tins Versus Cartons

It is now thought that eating food from tins rather than cartons can expose our bodies to more Bisphenol A (BPA) than would be the case with cartons. Many scientific studies have found links between BPA and serious health problems, from heart disease, diabetes and liver abnormalities in adults to developmental problems in the brains and hormonal systems of children.

For this reason it is better to choose cartons of food over tins where possible. For example cartons of cooked, chopped tomatoes or passata and cartons of coconut milk over the tinned versions.

Sugars

We hear a lot about the increasing amount of sugar in our diet. It's true that we are eating more sugar now than ever before and yet we are buying less bags of sugar. This means that it is making its way in to our food. Try and stick to the motto "if it is not real, it is not a meal".

If you do want to make your own dishes and want to use some sweetener then these are the better options available to you:

- Blackstrap molasses is a good source of iron, chromium and calcium. It has a rich malty flavour and is sweeter than sugar so you only need a little.
- Honey is also sweeter than sugar. Try and get honey that has been organically and locally produced to reap the full benefits.
- Date sugar - Made from dried dates. The fruit is dehydrated, then ground to produce the sugar. Retaining many of the nutritional benefits of dates, it has a rich sweet flavour. Unfortunately it doesn't melt or dissolve so it can be used as an addition to porridge and yogurt but not in cooking.
- Brown Rice Syrup is made from boiling brown rice. It can be used in cooking or as a condiment.
- Stevia is a very sweet sugar substitute made from the leaves of the stevia plant. You only need about 1 tea-spoon of stevia powder instead of a cup of sugar. It comes in a few different forms, liquid or powder. It can have a slightly bitter aftertaste so experiment.

- Pure Maple Syrup is a very natural product that is boiled down from the sap of the maple tree. Use maple syrup as you would honey. Try to avoid the brands with fructose added to bulk them out.

Whilst on the subject of sugar I would also recommend that you opt for lower sugar products such as low sugar but high fruit jam, low sugar and salt baked beans and low sugar and salt ketchup if you would normally have the traditional varieties of these products. Do not feel the need to introduce them to your diet now if they are not there already though.

Good Fats

Otherwise known as essential fatty acids, we need these fats in our diet throughout our lives. Cravings for fatty foods often mean that we are deficient in essential fatty acids. Oily fish, nuts and seeds help to lubricate joints, skin and the vagina. They also help keep cholesterol in check.

Keeping the amount of refined carbohydrates and sugary foods we eat in check is important to keep adrenal glands healthy. As we age and our natural levels of oestrogen reduce, we rely on our adrenal glands to produce oestrogen. If the adrenal glands are busy managing blood sugar fluctuations they cannot concentrate on oestrogen production.

- Reduce intake of sugary and refined carbohydrate foods and drinks such as chocolate, biscuits, cakes, sweets as well as white bread, potatoes and pasta.
- Reduce your intake of stimulants such as tea, coffee and chocolate.
- Increase the amount of fibre in your diet through vegetable consumption some fruit and change to whole grains such as wholemeal bread, brown pasta and brown rice.

Soy Sauce

There are now several types of soy sauce on the market. The most commonly available is bottles of 'soy sauce' which is made from wheat. You can now also buy:

- Reduced Salt Soy Sauce
- Tamari which is made without wheat
- Liquid Aminos which is made without gluten but with additional essential amino acids

Whilst the first three types are available in supermarkets you'll find liquid aminos and tamari also available in health food stores.

Phytoestrogens

Whilst on the subject of soy we must mention phyto-estrogens. Phytoestrogens are plant based oestrogens that can help boost our natural levels of oestrogen at a time when they are in natural decline. These are found in soy products (BUT ONLY FERMENETED ones such as tempeh, tofu, miso, natto, soy sauce NOT soy milk, yogurt etc), celery, fennel, liquorice, rhubarb and ginseng flaxseeds, legumes including chickpeas and lentils, garlic, parsley, brown rice and oats. Be careful to buy the right kind of soy based foods to reap the benefits of additional oestrogen in your diet.

Portion Sizing

Many people associate the menopause with weight gain but, as we get older, we actually need fewer calories. Eating the correct balance of macronutrients will help and you will find the diagram on the next page is very useful from that perspective.

Protein

Ensure you eat enough protein foods that contain the amino acid 'tryptophan'. You can find it in turkey, bananas, oats and legumes. Tryptophan helps manufacture the neurotransmitter serotonin. Serotonin helps moods and may help control sleep and appetite which can make you feel better in yourself.

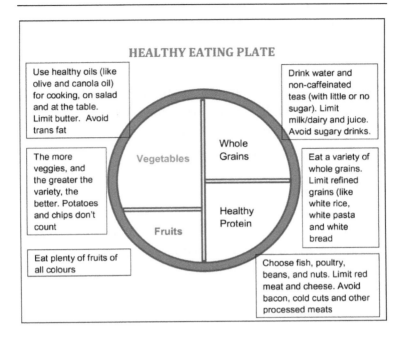

Source: Harvard School of Public Health

Which Fats To Cook With?

There is much discussion over which are the best fats to cook with and which should be left for dressings and dips. Here is a guide to make that whole subject easier to understand and follow:

- Saturated Fat, such as coconut oil, ghee and butter are ideal for cooking as the heat from cooking does not easily damage them or form free radicals.
- Polyunsaturated oils like sunflower, corn, soy or safflower should be strictly avoided for cooking as they are too easily damaged.

- Monounsaturated oils such as olive oil are fine up to a certain temperature i.e., no hotter than 180 degrees centigrade. Any higher than this then opt for a saturated fat such as coconut oil, butter or ghee.
- Meanwhile extra virgin olive oil (EVOO) should be kept for salad dressings and for dipping bread into. Good quality EVOO is quite expensive and should also be bottled in dark coloured glass to protect the delicate nutrients. Light and heat can both degrade the nutrient value of olive oil.

CHAPTER 5

MEAL IDEAS

Recipes for meal ideas with a '*' next to them can be found in chapters 6–10.

Breakfast

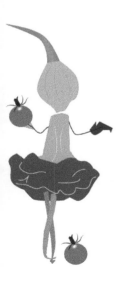

As a firm believer that a healthy breakfast really does set you up for the day, I wanted to share with you some ideas for junk-free break-fasts. The goal of a healthy breakfast is to make sure that your blood sugar levels do not peak and then trough half-way through the morning. If blood sugar levels stay more con-stant you're less likely to get irritable and more able to concentrate. Furthermore, breakfast is an opportunity to fuel your body with the nutrients that it needs. Here are some ideas for a healthy nutritious breakfast aimed at keeping your energy levels up long into the morning, and maybe even the afternoon.

- Wholemeal pancakes* or buckwheat pancakes* with natural yogurt, fresh or frozen berries and honey or maple syrup drizzled over.
- Poached eggs on rye toast.
- Protein packed porridge*.
- A 'grill-up' - grilled bacon, mushrooms, tomatoes and an egg (poached or scrambled).
- Mashed avocado on wholegrain or rye toast.
- Omelette with low sugar and salt baked beans.
- Sardines (½ tin of sardines in tomato sauce) on wholemeal or rye toast.
- Yogurt layers - take a glass or clear plastic cup. Layer natural yogurt with fresh fruit and low sugar granola or no added sugar muesli.
- Wholemeal bread roll with goats cheese and apricot jam (low sugar, high fruit such as St. Dalfour).
- Banana protein smoothie*.

Snacks

Snacking is by no means necessary but we often get caught short, far away from an ideal meal or just a little bit hungry. When we snack it is important to think about this as another opportunity to give your body the nutrients it needs. Here are some ideal snacks on the go:

- Nut butter* on apple slices.
- Nut butter* on wholesome oatcakes*.
- Spicy honey roasted seeds*.
- Soy sauce roasted seeds*.
- Red pepper hummus with crudités*.

- Celery with nut butter and cranberries*.

Quick Meals

- Ready to drink miso soup with rice noodles and cooked chicken or marinated tofu.
- Greek soup with courgettes, aubergines and feta*.
- Half an avocado and fresh prawns.
- Hummus and ready peeled and chopped crudités (carrots, peppers, cucumber) plus oatcakes or rice cakes if desired.
- Sun-dried tomatoes with ½ a tin of salmon or mackerel, ½ an avocado plus 2 Ryvita.
- Soft goats cheese with fresh figs and rocket on top of Ryvita.

Lunchtime meals

- Butternut squash falafel*.
- Spicy black bean turnovers*.
- Smoked tofu noodle soup*.
- Parsnip and apple soup*.
- Made-to-measure salad*
- Mackerel pate*.

Sides

- Roasted aubergine with oregano*.
- Cinnamon toasted butternut squash*.
- Carrot, raisin and almond salad*.
- Rocket salad with olive oil, salt and pepper.

Evening Meals

- Turkey and Apricot Burgers* with salad or roasted vegetables.
- Roasted red peppers with walnut and parsley pesto on wholegrain pasta*.
- Beef and lentil cottage pie*.
- Broccoli and broad bean frittata*.
- Sweet potato, goats cheese, red onion and baby spinach wholegrain pasta*.
- Spicy chicken dippers with roasted cauliflower and almond satay*.

Drinks

- Almond milk hot chocolate*.
- Rooibos tea.
- Green tea.
- Fennel tea.
- Peppermint tea.

Special Occasions

Banana bread*.

Chocolate and ginger fig truffles*.

CHAPTER 6

BREAKFAST RECIPES

Buckwheat Pancakes
(makes 20 small pancakes)

"Even my husband who is not a breakfast eater likes pancakes, especially these pancakes. You can always add a spoonful of maple syrup for a healthy treat." —Pat

Ingredients:

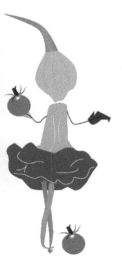

2 eggs

175g buckwheat flour

2 tsp baking powder

300ml milk

2 tbsp olive oil

Instructions:

Whisk the 2 eggs until light and frothy

Add the buckwheat flour and baking powder and mix again.

Add the milk and whisk well until you have a smooth batter with no lumps

Heat the olive oil in a wide frying pan

Drop a spoonful of the mixture into the pan

Watch carefully and turn when you see large bubbles at the edges of the pancakes.

Cook until golden brown on both sides.

Serve with a variety of toppings.

Wholemeal flour pancakes
(makes 8 pancakes)

Ingredients:

> 125g wholemeal flour or wholemeal spelt flour
>
> 1 medium egg
>
> 300ml milk

Instructions:

Place the flour in a large bowl, mix in the egg and gradually whisk in the milk to give a smooth batter.

Heat a little oil in a small frying pan and add a little of the batter to cover the base thinly.

Cook the pancake for 1 minute until golden, turn and cook for 30 seconds. Repeat.

Protein Packed Porridge
(serves 2 adults)

"I eat porridge most mornings. I am always looking for new things to add to make it tasty. This recipe fits the bill." —Pat

Ingredients:

100g (3 ½ oz) porridge oats (water to cover)

1 tbsp tahini

1 tbsp ground linseeds/flaxseeds

1 ripe banana (mashed)

1 tbsp honey

Instructions:

Put the oats and the water into a saucepan and cook gently until the porridge thickens up. Take the pan off the heat and stir all the other ingredients in.

Banana Protein Smoothie
(serves 4)

"This recipe is quick, easy and delicious. Peel the banana before you wrap it in in cling film and freeze it. I

can tell you from experience that it is not easy to peel a frozen banana!" —Pat

Ingredients:

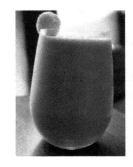

210g sliced frozen banana

20g protein powder

40g nut butter

250g almond milk

Instructions:

Put all ingredients into a food processor and whizz to combine.

CHAPTER 7

SNACK RECIPES

Wholesome Oatcakes
(makes 10 oatcakes)

"These oatcakes are simple to make and can be handy to add to your lunchbox if you are eating at work." —Pat

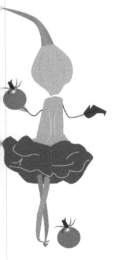

Ingredients:

    150g rolled oats

    10g butter

    125ml boiling water

    Sea salt

Instructions:

Preheat the oven to 180°C/350°F

Put the butter and salt in a bowl and pour over the boiling water. Stir to combine.

Add the oats and leave for 5 minutes.

Roll out dough on a floured surface and cut into about 10 oatcakes.

Bake for 8-10 minutes on a lightly greased baking sheet.

Cool on a wire rack.

Spicy Honey Roasted Seeds

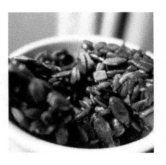

"I advise my weight loss clients to have a list of healthy treats that they can turn to if they feel peckish between meals. I would add these tasty seeds to that list" —Pat

Ingredients:

> 250g seeds (pumpkin and sunflower mixed)
>
> 3 tbsp honey
>
> 1 ½ tbsp olive oil or rice bran oil
>
> ½ tsp salt

Instructions:

Place all of the ingredients except the seeds into a saucepan and combine over a medium heat.

Add the seeds and stir until evenly coated.

Spread the seeds on a baking sheet lined with greaseproof paper.

Bake at 180°C/350°F for 20 minutes stirring once.

Leave to cool.

Enjoy immediately or store in the fridge in an airtight container.

Soy Sauce Roasted Seeds
(makes about 10 small portions)

Ingredients:

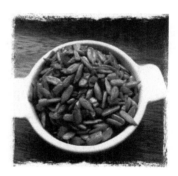

    125g sunflower seeds

    Olive oil to coat

    Soy sauce

Instructions:

Take the raw sunflower seeds and add a dash of olive oil and a dash of tamari soy sauce.

Stir the oil and the soy sauce into the sunflower seeds until covered then lay out flat on a baking sheet/tray:

Roast the sunflower seeds in a preheated oven at 180°C/350°F for about 15 minutes or until golden. Leave to cool before eating.

Red Pepper Hummus

"I am a big fan of hummus and often have it with salad and vegetable sticks for my lunch. This is a delicious variation." —Pat

Ingredients:

> 2 cloves of garlic, crushed
>
> 410g chickpeas, drained
>
> ½ 285g jar whole sweet red peppers, drained
>
> 1 tsp honey
>
> Tabasco, a few drops (optional)
>
> ½ tsp smoked paprika
>
> Black pepper

Instructions:

Put all of the ingredients (except black pepper) into the food processor and whizz until combined and hummus texture. Twist black pepper over the top before serving.

<u>Celery With Nut Butter And Cranberries</u>
(serves 4 as a snack)

"Jenny recently introduced me to nut butter and now I am a big fan. This recipe is a lovely combination of flavours." —Pat

Ingredients:

> 2 celery sticks
>
> 12 dried cranberries (ideally sweetened with fruit juice not sugar)
>
> Nut or seed butter (to fill the celery sticks)

Instructions:

Cut the celery into small sticks

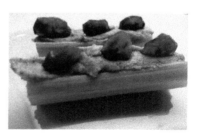

Fill the cavity with nut or seed butter.

Place the cranberries on top.

CHAPTER 8

QUICK MEALS AND LUNCH RECIPES

Greek Soup With Courgettes, Aubergines and Feta (serves 2)

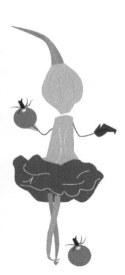

"During the winter I like my homemade soups for lunch. I might make an exception and eat this soup in the spring, summer and autumn as well!"
—Pat

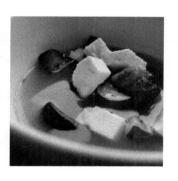

Ingredients:

  ½ aubergine in cubes

  1 courgette in cubes

  Olive oil

  Salt

½ pack Feta, cubed.

Vegetable bouillon made up to 180ml with water

Instructions:

Toss the chopped vegetables in olive oil. Sprinkle salt over them and put them onto a baking sheet in a pre-heated oven at 180°C/350°F.

Add the bouillon.

Heat all ingredients except the cheese in a saucepan.

Add the cheese at the very last minute.

Butternut Squash Falafel
(makes about 18 falafels)

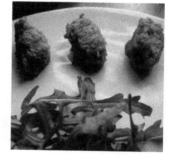

"I enjoy having these tasty falafels for lunch with salad. They are very useful for including in lunchboxes. I sometimes substitute ground coriander and cumin with the Moroccan mix of spices, ras al hanout." Pat

Ingredients:

> 400g cooked butternut squash (approximately one whole squash, peeled deseeded and cooked until soft)
>
> 100g chickpeas
>
> 2 tbsp gram flour
>
> ½ tsp ground coriander
>
> 1 tsp ground cumin
>
> Juice of ¼ lemon
>
> 2 tbsp olive oil or rice bran oil.

Instructions:

Put all ingredients into a food processor and whizz to combine to a smooth but thick paste.

Leave in a fridge for 24 hours

Make into small falafel balls.

Heat .the oil in a frying pan

Lightly fry the falafel until crispy on the outside but fluffy and sweet on the inside.

Drain using a piece of kitchen towel on a plate.

Spicy Black Bean Turnovers
(makes 8 turnovers)

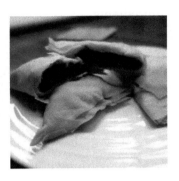

"This combination of flavours is right up my street. Eat them hot and then, if you can stop the rest of the family from eating them, you may have some leftover to eat cold."
—Pat

Ingredients:

> 200g roughly chopped brown onions
>
> 2 cloves of garlic, crushed
>
> 3 tbsp sun-dried tomato paste
>
> 1 tsp ground cumin
>
> ½ tsp ground cinnamon
>
> ½ tsp salt
>
> 400g tin of black beans, drained and rinsed thoroughly
>
> 6 sheets of filo pastry
>
> 1 tbsp olive oil plus some olive oil for brushing

Instructions:

Heat 1 tbsp olive oil in a medium saucepan.

Add the onions and crushed garlic.

Sweat the onion and garlic with the lid on for 10 minutes over a low heat.

Add the spices and tomato paste. Allow the flavours to merge then add the black beans and salt.

Gently mash the black beans into the other ingredients with a fork or potato masher.

When cooked through remove from the heat.

Lay out your filo pastry sheets and chop the sheets into 8 squares.

Brush the perimeter of the squares layered 2-3 sheets at a time) with olive oil. Pop a dollop of the blackbean mix in one half and fold over to make a triangle.

Brush the top of the turnover with olive oil.

Place the turnovers on a baking tray that you have brushed with olive oil too.

Bake at 180°C/ 350°F for about 15 minutes or until they are crispy. Enjoy hot or cold.

Parsnip And Apple Soup
(serves 4)

"This for me is a classic autumn soup. The spices are optional but I enjoy the depth of flavour they bring to the soup." —Pat

Ingredients:

700g parsnips, peeled and cubed

1 cooking apple, cored and grated

1 tbsp olive oil

2 medium onions, chopped

2 cloves garlic, crushed

Spices (optional): 1 heaped tsp ground ginger, 1 tsp cumin and 1 tsp turmeric

1 litre vegetable stock

Salt and pepper

Instructions:

Heat the oil in a pan and cook the onions for 2 minutes.

Add the crushed garlic and cook for a further 1 minute before adding the spices.

Stir and then add the parsnips, stock and seasoning (salt, pepper and spices if using).

Stir and let the soup simmer.

Remove from the heat and then liquidize.

Return to the heat and just as the soup reaches simmering point add the grated apple.

Simmer for a few more minutes, then serve or allow the soup to cool before storing in the fridge.

Smoked Tofu Noodle Soup
(serves 2)

"The good thing about tofu, apart from the many health benefits, is the way that it soaks up the flavours of this soup. If left in the fridge the noodles soak up the liquid and make a delicious noodle dish, simply reheat" —Pat

Ingredients:

- 1 clove garlic, crushed
- 1 onion, chopped
- 1 tbsp. olive oil
- 1 pack smoked tofu, copped into 2cm squares
- 3 carrots, diced
- 575ml vegetable stock or 1 stock cube and 575ml water
- Rice noodles (100g per person)

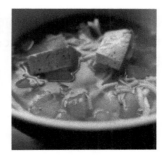

Instructions:

In a medium saucepan sauté the onion for 2 minutes then add the garlic. Saute for a further minute

Add the carrots and the stock to the saucepan. Cover and simmer for about 15 minutes.

Meanwhile bring another saucepan of water to the boil. Add the rice noodles and cook for 5 minutes, until soft and ready to eat.

Drain, rinse (to get rid of excess starch) then add the noodles and the chopped tofu to the carrot soup pot. Heat through and then serve half immediately.

Made-to-Measure Salads

Step 1: Pick your leaves—rocket, watercress, baby spinach, romaine

Step 2: Add some salad vegetables—tomato, cucumber, grated carrot, radish, broccoli, peppers, red onion, olives, avocado, beetroot, mushrooms

Step 3: Decide on protein—kidney beans, chick peas, tuna, salmon, egg, cheese, cottage cheese, edamame beans

Step 4: A bit of crunch—seeds (sunflower, sesame, pumpkin, chia), nuts (any), croutons (garlic, plain, gluten free, polenta), crispy bacon

Step 5: Just a handful of carbohydrates—noodles, pasta, rice, new potatoes in their skins, tortilla chips, pitta chips

Step 6: Pick a dressing—Italian, French, Oriental, Honey and Mustard

Dressings:

With each of the following recipes for salad dressings simply combine the ingredients in the order suggested.

1. <u>Italian</u>
(makes about 150ml)

Ingredients:

125ml olive oil

3 ½ tbsp. balsamic vinegar

2 tbsp grated Parmesan

Freshly ground black pepper

¾ tsp salt

¼ tsp garlic powder

2. French
(makes about 120ml)

Ingredients:

  90ml extra virgin olive oil

  1tbsp white wine vinegar

  1 tsp French mustard

  Pinch sugar

3. Oriental
(makes about 6Tbsp)

Ingredients:

  Grated rind and juice of 2 limes (roll on a surface
    first to get the most juice out)

  2 tbsp Thai fish sauce

  2 tbsp unrefined sugar

  2 small garlic cloves, crushed

  2 lemon grass stalks finely sliced

  1 fresh chilli, finely chopped (optional)

4. Honey and Mustard
(makes about 180ml)

Ingredients:

  6tbsp Dijon mustard

3 tbsp honey

60ml olive oil

1-2 tsp lemon juice

½ tsp garlic powder

¼ tsp ground black pepper

5. **<u>Mustard and Linseed Vinaigrette</u>**
(makes about 250ml)

Ingredients:

1 clove of garlic crushed

1 tbsp finely chopped shallots

1 tsp caster sugar

½ tsp salt

Some freshly ground black pepper

½ teaspoon dried herbs of Provence

1 tsp English mustard

150ml The Linseed Farm Culinary Linseed Oil

40ml white wine vinegar or cider vinegar

40ml lemon juice

CHAPTER 9

SIDES RECIPES

Aubergine With Oregano
(serves 2 as a side dish)

"This dish goes well with fish or chicken."
—Pat

Ingredients:

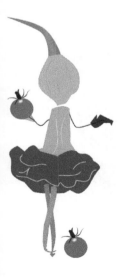

    1 large or 2 medium aubergines

    2 tbsps of olive oil

    A pinch of dry oregano

    Salt and pepper to taste

Instructions:

Pre-heat the oven to 200°C/390°F

Dice the aubergine(s) into rough chunks and place in a roasting pan

Sprinkle with oregano and salt and pepper

Pour over the olive oil

Bake in the pre-heated oven for 30 minutes until soft

Cinnamon Toasted Butternut Squash
(serves 4 as a side dish)

"This is such a simple and tasty recipe. A good dish for lunchtime or as a side dish for supper." —Pat

Ingredients:

    1 medium sized butternut squash

    2 tbsp of olive oil

    Salt

    1 tsp of Cinnamon powder

Instructions:

Pre heat oven to
180°C/3560°F

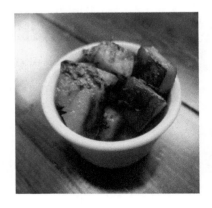

Chop the squash into cubes and place in a roasting pan.

Sprinkle over salt and cinnamon and add a good glug of olive oil

Roast in the pre-heated oven for 20-30 minutes until soft.

Carrot, Raisin And Almond Salad
(serves 2 as a small salad)

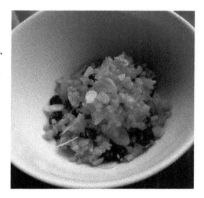

"I love the flavours of Moroccan salads and this recipe reminds me of some lovely meals in Marrakesh." —Pat

Ingredients;

    1 large carrot

    A handful of raisins

    A handful of flaked almonds

    Olive oil

    Balsamic vinegar

    Salt and pepper

Instructions

Grate the carrot by hand or in a food processor.

Add a handful of raisins and a handful of flaked almonds.

Then add a glug of olive oil and a glug of balsamic vinegar.

Add a twist of salt and pepper and you have a very simple side salad.

CHAPTER 10

EVENING MEALS

Turkey and Apricot Burgers
(makes 8 small burgers)

"I first had the combination of turkey and apricots in a salad in Bath many years ago. This recipe brings back those flavours and some happy memories." —Pat

Ingredients:

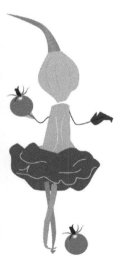

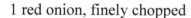

 1 red onion, finely chopped

 1 tsp olive oil

 225g minced turkey

 1 organic eating apple, grated

 2 tsp. low sugar apricot jam

 2 medium potatoes, cooked and then mashed

Sesame seeds

Instructions:

In a saucepan heat the oil and sauté the onions until soft.

Add the turkey mince and cook, stirring constantly until cooked through.

Take off the heat and mix in the remaining ingredients then allow to rest and cool.

When cool form small burgers in your hands. Pop these in the fridge for 30 minutes.

Brush with olive oil and then coat in sesame seeds.

Grill for about 7 minutes on a low-medium heat.

Roasted Pepper Pesto On Wholegrain Pasta
(serves 4)

"I particularly like this with avocado slices and a fresh green salad." —Pat

Ingredients:

    1 x 285g jar roasted red peppers in oil

    50g walnuts

    8 cloves garlic, peeled

    1 bunch parsley

    60ml of oil from red pepper jar (make up with olive oil if not enough)

Black pepper

Wholewheat penne, large handful (dried) per person

Instructions:

Drain the red peppers, keeping the oil, and put the red peppers to one side.

Whizz together walnuts, garlic and parsley in a food processor. Drizzle in the oil while the blade is turning to form a thick pesto paste.

Add black pepper to taste.

Stir into freshly cooked wholewheat penne pasta.

Lay the red peppers on top.

Beef And Lentil Cottage Pie
(serves 4)

"This is a useful recipe if you want to include some red meat in your diet but keep it healthy. I sometimes substitute sweet potatoes for the mash." —Pat

Ingredients:

250g lean mined beef

1 large onion, chopped

150g dry green lentils, rinsed

400g chopped tomatoes

4 carrots, diced

150g frozen peas

200ml beef stock

2 tbsp tomato ketchup

For the mash:

1kg potatoes, peeled and chopped

25g butter

3 tbsp almond milk

Instructions:

Preheat the oven to 180°C/375°F

Put the mince and onions in a large saucepan and cook until the mince has browned.

Add the remaining ingredients and cook for about 30 minutes until the lentils and vegetables are soft. Add a little water if necessary.

Pour into an ovenproof dish.

Meanwhile boil the potatoes until tender. Drain and mash them, adding the butter and enough almond milk to make a soft mash.

Place the mash on top of the beef and lentil mix and spread evenly.

Pop this dish in the oven for 30 minutes until the top is golden brown.

Broccoli And Broad Bean Frittata
(serves2)

"We all know that broccoli and kale are good for us and they are absolutely delicious in this recipe!" —Pat

Ingredients:

20g butter

1 medium onion, sliced

110g potatoes, boiled and sliced

80g broccoli florets, cooked

25g kale, cooked

80g broad beans, cooked

4 eggs

Salt and pepper.

Instructions:

Melt the butter in a frying pan. Add the onion and sauté.

Add the potato and cook until golden brown. Add the remaining vegetables and heat through.

Finally add the eggs (beaten with salt and pepper).

Leave to set for a minute or so then cook under a grill for a further 1 minute until the top is golden brown.

Serve.

Goats Cheese, Sweet Potato, Red Onion and Baby Spinach Wholegrain Pasta

(serves4)

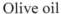

Ingredients:

> 2 sweet potatoes, peeled and chopped into 2cm squares
>
> Olive oil
>
> Salt
>
> 1 red onion, finely sliced
>
> ½ pack baby spinach, washed and ready to use
>
> 1 pack soft goat's cheese, cubed
>
> Wholegrain pasta, large handful (dried) per person.

Instructions:

Pre-heat the oven to 180°C/3760°F

Roast sweet potato cubes in olive oil and a pinch of salt for 20 minutes, until soft. Turn once or twice.

Sauté the onions in olive oil, at a very low heat, for about 20 minutes. With the lid on they will become 1 soft and sweet.

Bring a pan of water to the boil. Add the pasta and cook until al dente.

When the pasta is ready add the baby spinach to the pasta pan for 30-40 seconds then drain.

Add the cooked sweet potato, cooked onions and then the goat's cheese to the pasta. Heat and stir until combined. Serve.

Spicy Chicken Dippers With Roasted Cauliflower And Almond Satay (serves 4)

"This is a straightforward recipe that is packed with taste. You can eat the dippers on their own but I love the nutty dip." —Pat

Ingredients for the chicken dippers:

- 3 free range chicken breasts, sliced
- 2 tbsps soy sauce
- 1 ½ tsp ground coriander
- 1 tsp ground cumin
- 1 tbsp olive oil

Instructions for the chicken dippers:

Season the chicken with the soy sauce, olive oil and spices. Make sure all the chicken slices are completely covered.

Grill for about 4-5 minutes each side, until the chicken is cooked through but still moist..

Ingredients for the roasted cauliflower:

- 1 cauliflower head chopped into small florets, washed
- 1 tbsp turmeric
- 2 tbsp olive oil
- Good pinch sea salt

Instructions for the roasted cauliflower:

Combine the olive oil and turmeric and coat the cauliflower with this mixture

Sprinkle with salt and pop into the oven at 180°C/350°F for 20-25 minutes, tossing once or twice during the cooking process.

Ingredients for the almond satay:

- 3 tbsp almond butter
- 2 tbsp coconut milk

2 tbsp warm water

1 garlic clove, crushed,

1 tbsp fresh root ginger, finely chopped

1 tsp soy sauce

2 tsp of olive oil

1 tsp fish sauce

Instructions for the almond satay:

Put all of the ingredients into a food processor and whizz together.

Smoked Mackerel Pate
(serves 4)

"My husband and I like smoked mackerel pate as a starter or as light evening meal with some salad and wholemeal toast." —Pat

Ingredients:

300g smoked mackerel fillets

200g probiotic Greek yogurt

2 tbsp creamed horseradish

1 lemon

Ground black pepper

Instructions:

Peel the skin off the mackerel fillets.

Put into a blender with 100g of the yogurt, the juice of the lemon and some black pepper and horseradish.

Blend until smooth then add the last 100g yogurt but stir slowly.

CHAPTER 11

SPECIAL OCCASION RECIPES

Almond Milk Hot Chocolate

Warm a cup of almond milk on the hob to a simmer. Pour hot milk over 3 squares of 70% cocoa solids dark chocolate and stir to combine.

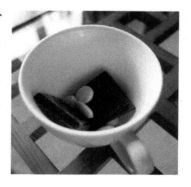

Banana Bread

"I am not a natural cake maker but even I can make this bread. It is always lovely and moist and great spread with a little butter." —Pat

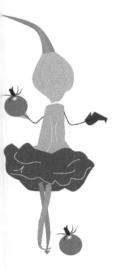

Ingredients:

Wet Ingredients

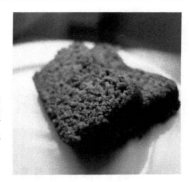

- 1 tbsp ground linseeds (flaxseeds) mixed with 3 tbsp warm water
- 4 ripe bananas
- 75g soft butter, plus extra for greasing and serving
- 1 tsp vanilla extract

Dry Ingredients

- 170g) spelt flour
- 120g unrefined sugar
- 1 tsp bicarbonate of soda
- 1 pinch of salt

Instructions:

Preheat the oven to 180C/350°F

Grease a 30 x 23-cm loaf tin. Line with a cross pattern of two strips of greaseproof paper to make the cake easy to extract from the tin when baked.

Make up the ground flaxseeds and water mix and allow to stand. Mash the bananas either by hand or using a food processor.

Add to the banana the flaxseeds and water mix and then add the butter and vanilla extract. Mix together.

In a separate bowl mix the dry ingredients.

Combine the two.

Pour into the greased and lined loaf tin.

Bake for 1 hour.

Leave to cool and remove from the tin and then allow to cool a little more on a cooling rack.

Enjoy warm or cold and with or without butter.

Chocolate and Ginger Fig Truffles

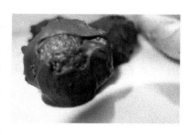

"Jenny knows that I love ginger so she included this recipe for me. Ginger is anti-inflammatory and may provide relief from migraine. A healthy reason to eat chocolate." —Pat

Ingredients:

> 350g dried figs (the soft and gooey ones) with stalks removed
>
> 155g crystalized ginger

½ tsp ground cinnamon

Pinch nutmeg

Pinch ground cloves

85g bar dark chocolate

Instructions:

Put the figs, ginger and spices into a food processor and whizz until combined. This may take up to a minute to break the ginger down.

Once whizzed, mould the mixture into table tennis sized balls using the palms of your hands.

Place the balls on a sheet of grease proof paper on a plate in the fridge whilst you melt the chocolate.

Melt the broken chocolate in a bowl over boiling water being careful to ensure the bowl doesn't touch the water. Once melted roll the cold fig balls in the chocolate to coat.

Place the truffles back into the fridge and wait for an hour.

Appendix A:

MENOPAUSE SYMPTOMS RECORD

Use the following table to keep a record of any menopausal symptoms that you are experiencing and anything that you have become aware of that triggers the symptom. You may also want to keep a note of the stage in your menstrual cycle when you experience the symptom.

You can access the following bonus products at
www.hotwomencoolsolutions.com

Symptom	Yes/No	Frequency (per day or per week)	Intensity (scale of 1 to 5)
Tension			
Mood swings			
Depression			
Forgetfulness			
Poor or interrupted sleep			
Weight change			
Headache			
Tiredness			
Dizziness or faintness			
Heart pounding			
Hot flush			
Night sweat			
Irregular periods			
Heavier/lighter periods			
Breast tenderness			
Abdominal bloating			

- The Menopause workbook including: Menopausal Symptoms Journal, Sleep Journal, Food Journal, Faulty Thinking Journal and Positivity Journal
- Change Happens—Top Tips for Succeeding in Challenging Times
- Stay Cool Hypnotic Relaxation Recording
- Mindful Weight Loss Hypnotic Relaxation Recording
- Sleep Well—Always! Hypnotic Relaxation Recording

See more at:
http://hotwomencoolsolutions.com/bonuses/?action=subscribed#sthash.syPbvo3L.dpuf

APPENDIX B:

WEEKLY MENU PLAN

With the template on the following pages you can plan your meals for the week to ensure that you get all of the nutrition your body requires. You can use the plan as the basis for your weekly shopping list.

Columns Key:
Carb = unrefined carbohydrates
P = protein
Calc = calcium
F = fruit
V = vegetables
D = drink

	Carb	P	Calc	F	V	D
Example; Red pepper hummus and whole-meal toast	x	x	x		x	
Monday						
Breakfast						
Lunch						
Dinner						
Tuesday						
Breakfast						
Lunch						
Dinner						
Wednesday						
Breakfast						

Lunch						
Dinner						
Thursday						
Breakfast						
Lunch						
Dinner						
Friday						
Breakfast						
Lunch						
Dinner						
Saturday						

Breakfast						
Lunch						
Dinner						
Sunday						
Breakfast						
Lunch						
Dinner						

Appendix C:

RECIPES BY SYMPTOM

For Hot Flushes

Protein Packed Porridge

Spicy Honey Roasted Seeds

Soy Sauce Roasted Seeds

Red Pepper Hummus

Greek Soup with courgettes, aubergines and feta

Butternut squash falafel

Spicy Black Bean Turnovers

Smoked Tofu Noodle Soup

Linseed Vinaigrette

Broccoli and broad bean frittata

Spicy Chicken Dippers with roasted cauliflower and almond satay

For Healthy Bowels

Protein Packed Porridge

Banana Protein Smoothie

Wholesome Oatcakes

Spicy Honey Roasted Seeds

Soy Sauce Roasted Seeds

Red pepper hummus

Instant Greek Soup with courgettes, aubergines and feta

Butternut squash falafel

Spicy Black Bean Turnovers

Made-to-Measure Salads

Aubergine with oregano

Cinnamon Toasted Butternut Squash

Carrot, Raisin and Almond salad

Beef and Lentil Cottage Pie

Broccoli and broad bean frittata

Chocolate and Ginger Fig Truffles

For Strong Bones

Banana Protein Smoothie

Soy Sauce Roasted Seeds

Greek Soup with courgettes, aubergines and feta

Smoked Tofu Noodle Soup

Carrot, Raisin and Almond salad

Turkey and Apricot Burgers

Broccoli and broad bean frittata

Goats cheese, sweet potato, spinach and pasta

Almond Milk Hot Chocolate

Banana Bread

For a Happy Heart

Buckwheat pancakes

Wholemeal flour pancakes

Banana Protein Smoothie

Wholesome Oatcakes

Soy Sauce Roasted Seeds

Red Pepper Hummus

Instant Greek Soup with courgettes, aubergines and feta

Spicy Black Bean Turnovers

Smoked Tofu Noodle Soup

Aubergine with oregano

Cinnamon Toasted Butternut Squash

Cinnamon Toasted Butternut Squash

Carrot, Raisin and Almond salad

Roasted red peppers with walnut and parsley pesto on wholegrain pasta

Broccoli and broad bean frittata

Goats cheese, sweet potato, red onion and baby spinach wholegrain pasta

Banana Bread

Chocolate and Ginger Fig Truffles

For Good Mood

Banana Protein Smoothie

Spicy Black Bean Turnovers

Carrot, Raisin and Almond salad

Roasted red peppers with walnut and parsley pesto on wholegrain pasta

Smoked Mackerel Pate

Almond Milk Hot Chocolate

Banana Bread

Chocolate and Ginger Fig Truffles

For Hair, Skin and Nails

Buckwheat pancakes

Wholemeal flour pancakes

Soy Sauce Roasted Seeds

Made-to-Measure Salad

Cinnamon Toasted Butternut Squash

Carrot, Raisin and Almond salad

Roasted red peppers with walnut and parsley pesto on wholegrain pasta

Broccoli and broad bean frittata

Smoked Mackerel Pate

Almond Milk Hot Chocolate

For Healthy Breasts

Buckwheat pancakes

Wholesome Oatcakes

Spicy Black Bean Turnover

Smoked Tofu Noodle Soup

Cinnamon Toasted Butternut Squash

Broccoli and broad bean frittata

Weight Control

Made-to-Measure Salads

Smoked Tofu Noodle Soup

Aubergine with oregano

Carrot, Raisin and Almond salad

Turkey and Apricot Burgers

Spicy Chicken Dippers with roasted cauliflower and almond satay

Smoked Mackerel Pate

Almond Milk Hot Chocolate

APPENDIX D:

RESOURCES

Elements for Life Online supplier of nut milk bags, raw chocolate and ingredients

http://www.elementsforlife.co.uk/

Coldfront A personal cooling kit for hot flushes

http://www.mycoldfront.com/

Goodness Direct Online Health Food Store

http://www.goodnessdirect.co.uk/cgi-local/frameset/script/home.html

Hot Women Cool Solutions Blogs, advice and tips for controlling menopause symptoms

www.hotwomencoolsolutions.com

Lunchbox Doctor for menu plans and recipes

http://www.lunchboxdoctor.com/

Natural Health Practice Suppliers of vitamins and minerals

http://www.naturalhealthpractice.com/

Pampered Chef Direct seller of high quality kitchen tools

http://www.pamperedchef.co.uk/

Thermomix Multi-functional kitchen appliance and all-in-one cooking system

http://thermomix.vorwerk.co.uk/

The Linseed Farm Suppliers of linseed products, advice and recipes

http://thelinseedfarm.co.uk/

Vevie Active leisure wear in flattering styles and in fabrics that allow your skin to breathe

www.vevie.com

Useful Websites

Continence

ACA Association for Continence Advice

www.aca.uk.com

ACPWH Association of Chartered Physiotherapists in Women's Health

www.womentsphysio.com

Hypertension

American Society for Hypertension

www.ash-us.org/

British Hypertension Society

www.bhsoc.org/default.stm

Hypnotension TM—complementary approach to tackling high blood pressure:

www.hypnotension.com/

NHS UK

http://www.nhs.uk/conditions/Blood-pressure-(high)/Pages/Introduction.aspx

Hysterectomy

Hysterectomy

www.hysterectomyconsequences.com

Osteoporosis

NHS UK

www.nhs.uk/Conditions/Osteoporosis/Pages/Introduction.aspx

National Osteoporosis Society in UK

www.nos.org.uk/

National Osteoporosis Foundation USA

www.nof.org/

Perimenopause

UK
www.nhs.uk/Conditions/Menopause/Pages/Introduction.aspx

US
www.WebMD.com/menopause

US
www.fda.gov/womens/menopause

General Menopause Websites

For up to date advice and resources
www.shmirshky.com

The Change Explained
https://www.facebook.com/TheChangeExplained

The North American Menopause Society
www.menopause.org/

Information about symptoms and treatment options
www.menopausematters.co.uk/

Appendix E:

REFERENCES

Glenville, Marilyn (1997) Natural alternatives to HRT, Kyle Cathie Ltd

Goldman, Mindy, MD, (2010)
www.breastcancer.org/tips/menopausal/ask_expert/2004
_07/queston_04

ABOUT THE AUTHORS

Pat Duckworth MBA, NLP Master Prac., Dip CHyp., HPD., is a Cognitive Hypnotherapist, award winning author and trainer.

Pat sees clients on a one-to-one basis at her therapy rooms in Harley Street, London, Cambridgeshire and Toronto. She specialises in helping women experiencing menopause symptoms including hot flushes, weight gain, poor sleep, loss of confidence and mood swings.

Pat has designed and delivered training and workshops on a wide range of well-being subjects and is a sought after public-speaker. She is a regular guest on BBC Radio Cambridgeshire. She has had a series of articles published by The Hypnotherapy Journal.

In 2012 she published 'Hot Women, Cool Solutions; How to control menopause symptoms using mind/body techniques', followed by 'How to Survive Her Menopause; A practical guide to women's health for men' in 2013. She has also contributed to 'Your 101 Ways to 101' by Dr George Grant and 'The Planet of Wellness' by Marina Nani.

Pat is a consultant to the CAM Fertility Centre and to the Active Mum programme

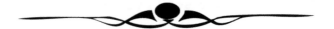

Jenny Tschiesche (BSc(Hons) Dip(ION) FdSc BANT) is one of the UK's leading nutrition experts, award winning author and founder of wwwlunchboxdoctor.com.

With an international reputation and following, Jenny is an expert in all fields of nutrition. She provides specialist nutrition and dietary advice to a wide range of people including top athletes, sporting bodies, people dealing with illness and parents and their children. Jenny has a clinic in Marlow, Bucks

Jenny is also a naturally gifted and inspirational public speaker having conducted many public and corporate workshops, seminars, event and talks to audiences from small intimate numbers to 1000s at a time. With many years' experience in the field of nutrition Jenny can speak and advise on a very wide range of health-related subjects including: weight management, women's health, child nutrition, sports nutrition, allergies and intolerances.

Jenny regularly contributes to national Radio, TV, press and social media coverage including:

- 5 Live
- Sky News
- The Guardian
- The Daily Telegraph
- Channel 4 News
- Zest
- Men's Health
- Healthy Magazine
- The Mail
- The Express
- BBC Radio
- Prima
- Top Sante

Lightning Source UK Ltd.
Milton Keynes UK
UKHW021818251021
392832UK00006B/209